THE BOOK BELONGS TO:

_____

_____

_____

_____

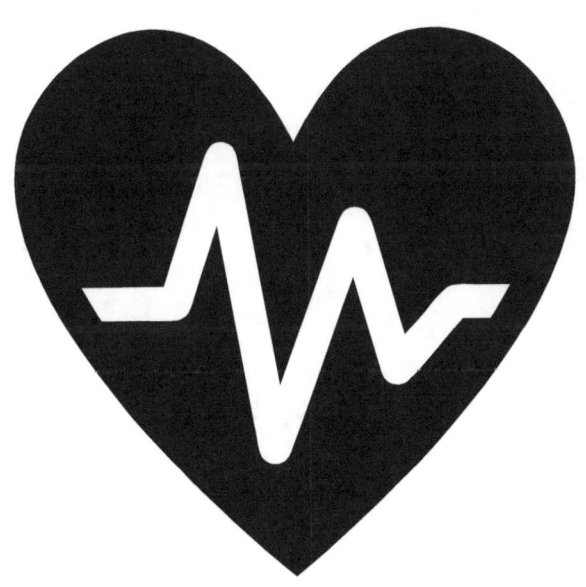

TABLE OF CONTENTS

CONTENT	PAGE
Personal Information	1
Emergency Contacts	1
Insurance Information	2
Pharmacy Information	2
My Medical Quick View	3
Medical Conditions	3
Allergies	3
Medications List	4-5
Surgical History	6-7
Family Medical History	8-11
Notes	12-13
My Medical Tests/Procedures	14-63

MEDICAL TEST/PROCEDURES
TABLE OF CONTENTS

TEST/PROCEDURE	DATE	PAGE

MEDICAL TEST/PROCEDURES
TABLE OF CONTENTS

TEST/PROCEDURE	DATE	PAGE

MEDICAL TEST/PROCEDURES
TABLE OF CONTENTS

TEST/PROCEDURE	DATE	PAGE

MEDICAL TEST/PROCEDURES
TABLE OF CONTENTS

TEST/PROCEDURE	DATE	PAGE

MEDICAL TEST/PROCEDURES
TABLE OF CONTENTS

TEST/PROCEDURE	DATE	PAGE

MEDICAL TEST/PROCEDURES
TABLE OF CONTENTS

TEST/PROCEDURE	DATE	PAGE

PERSONAL INFORMATION

Name: _____

Address: _____ City: _____

State/Zip: _____ Home Ph #: _____

Work Ph #: _____ Cell Ph # _____

EMERGENCY CONTACTS:

Name: _____

Address: _____ City: _____

State/Zip: _____ Home Ph #: _____

Work Ph #: _____ Cell Ph # _____

Relationship: _____

Name: _____

Address: _____ City: _____

State/Zip: _____ Home Ph #: _____

Work Ph #: _____ Cell Ph # _____

Relationship: _____

Name: _____

Address: _____ City: _____

State/Zip: _____ Home Ph #: _____

Work Ph #: _____ Cell Ph # _____

Relationship: _____

INSURANCE & PHARMACY

Insurance Company:

Plan Type: _____ Policyholder : _____

Group #: _____ ID #: _____

Phone # : _____ Website: _____

Username: _____ Password: _____

Insurance Company:

Plan Type: _____ Policyholder : _____

Group #: _____ ID #: _____

Phone # : _____ Website: _____

Username: _____ Password: _____

Insurance Company:

Plan Type: _____ Policyholder : _____

Group #: _____ ID #: _____

Phone # : _____ Website: _____

Username: _____ Password: _____

PHARMACY INFORMATION

Name:	Name:
Phone:	Phone:
Fax:	Fax:
Location:	Location:

MY MEDICAL QUICK VIEW

Name: _____ Donor: Y / N _____

Date of Birth: _____ Blood Type: _____

Height: _____ Weight: _____

MEDICAL CONDITIONS:

- High Blood Pressure   YES / NO   MEDS: _____
- Diabetic   YES / NO   Insulin / Oral Meds / Both
- _____
- _____
- _____
- _____
- _____
- _____
- _____
- _____
- _____

ALLERGIES	REACTION	MEDICATION

MEDICATIONS

MEDS	DOSE	FREQUENCY	CONDITION	PHYSICIAN

MEDICATIONS

MEDS	DOSE	FREQUENCY	CONDITION	PHYSICIAN

SURGICAL HISTORY

SURGERY	DATE	FACILITY	ORDERING PHYSICIAN	SURGEON

SURGICAL HISTORY

SURGERY	DATE	FACILITY	ORDERING PHYSICIAN	SURGEON

FAMILY MEDICAL HISTORY

LIST FAMILY MEMBER IN TOP ROW

MEDICAL CONDITION				
High Blood Pressure				
Diabetes				
High Cholesterol				
Heart Disease				
Stroke/TIA				
Allergies				
Auto Immune Diseases				
Cancer				
Arthritis				
Birth Defects				
Infertility				
Mental Illness				
Kidney Disease				
Liver Disease				
Lung Disease				
Blood Disorder				
Gastrointestinal Disorder				
Muscular Diseases				
Nerve Disorders				
Skin Disorders				
Migraines				
Ocular Disease				
Epilepsy				
Endometriosis				

FAMILY MEDICAL HISTORY

			NOTES

FAMILY MEDICAL HISTORY

LIST FAMILY MEMBER IN TOP ROW

MEDICAL CONDITION				
High Blood Pressure				
Diabetes				
High Cholesterol				
Heart Disease				
Stroke/TIA				
Allergies				
Auto Immune Diseases				
Cancer				
Arthritis				
Birth Defects				
Infertility				
Mental Illness				
Kidney Disease				
Liver Disease				
Lung Disease				
Blood Disorder				
Gastrointestinal Disorder				
Muscular Diseases				
Nerve Disorders				
Skin Disorders				
Migraines				
Ocular Disease				
Epilepsy				
Endometriosis				

FAMILY MEDICAL HISTORY

			NOTES

NOTES

NOTES

MY MEDICAL TESTS/PROCEDURES

Facility:	Contact Person:
Address:	Phone:

Ordering Physician:

Test/Exam Ordered:

Duration:	Do I Need A Driver? YES / NO

Symptoms:

Appt. Date:	Arrival Time ___:___	Exam Time ___:___

Prep For Test:

Results:

Facility:	Contact Person:
Address:	Phone:

Ordering Physician:

Test/Exam Ordered:

Duration:	Do I Need A Driver? YES / NO

Symptoms:

Appt. Date:	Arrival Time ___:___	Exam Time ___:___

Prep For Test:

Results:

MY MEDICAL TESTS/PROCEDURES

Facility: | Contact Person:

Address: | Phone:

Ordering Physician:

Test/Exam Ordered:

Duration: | Do I Need A Driver? YES / NO

Symptoms:

Appt. Date: | Arrival Time ___:___ | Exam Time ___:___

Prep For Test:

Results:

Facility: | Contact Person:

Address: | Phone:

Ordering Physician:

Test/Exam Ordered:

Duration: | Do I Need A Driver? YES / NO

Symptoms:

Appt. Date: | Arrival Time ___:___ | Exam Time ___:___

Prep For Test:

Results:

MY MEDICAL TESTS/PROCEDURES

Facility:	Contact Person:
Address:	Phone:
Ordering Physician:	
Test/Exam Ordered:	
Duration:	Do I Need A Driver? YES / NO
Symptoms:	

Appt. Date: Arrival Time ___:___   Exam Time ___:___

Prep For Test:

Results:

Facility:	Contact Person:
Address:	Phone:
Ordering Physician:	
Test/Exam Ordered:	
Duration:	Do I Need A Driver? YES / NO
Symptoms:	

Appt. Date: Arrival Time ___:___   Exam Time ___:___

Prep For Test:

Results:

MY MEDICAL TESTS/PROCEDURES

Facility:	Contact Person:
Address:	Phone:

Ordering Physician:

Test/Exam Ordered:

Duration:	Do I Need A Driver? YES / NO

Symptoms:

Appt. Date:	Arrival Time ___:___	Exam Time ___:___

Prep For Test:

Results:

Facility:	Contact Person:
Address:	Phone:

Ordering Physician:

Test/Exam Ordered:

Duration:	Do I Need A Driver? YES / NO

Symptoms:

Appt. Date:	Arrival Time ___:___	Exam Time ___:___

Prep For Test:

Results:

MY MEDICAL TESTS/PROCEDURES

Facility: Contact Person:

Address: Phone:

Ordering Physician:

Test/Exam Ordered:

Duration: Do I Need A Driver? YES / NO

Symptoms:

Appt. Date: Arrival Time ___:___   Exam Time ___:___

Prep For Test:

Results:

Facility: Contact Person:

Address: Phone:

Ordering Physician:

Test/Exam Ordered:

Duration: Do I Need A Driver? YES / NO

Symptoms:

Appt. Date: Arrival Time ___:___   Exam Time ___:___

Prep For Test:

Results:

MY MEDICAL TESTS/PROCEDURES

Facility:	Contact Person:
Address:	Phone:
Ordering Physician:	
Test/Exam Ordered:	
Duration:	Do I Need A Driver? YES / NO
Symptoms:	

Appt. Date:	Arrival Time ___:___	Exam Time ___:___

Prep For Test:

Results:

Facility:	Contact Person:
Address:	Phone:
Ordering Physician:	
Test/Exam Ordered:	
Duration:	Do I Need A Driver? YES / NO
Symptoms:	

Appt. Date:	Arrival Time ___:___	Exam Time ___:___

Prep For Test:

Results:

MY MEDICAL TESTS/PROCEDURES

Facility: Contact Person:

Address: Phone:

Ordering Physician:

Test/Exam Ordered:

Duration: Do I Need A Driver? YES / NO

Symptoms:

Appt. Date: Arrival Time ___:___   Exam Time ___:___

Prep For Test:

Results:

Facility: Contact Person:

Address: Phone:

Ordering Physician:

Test/Exam Ordered:

Duration: Do I Need A Driver? YES / NO

Symptoms:

Appt. Date: Arrival Time ___:___   Exam Time ___:___

Prep For Test:

Results:

MY MEDICAL TESTS/PROCEDURES

Facility:	Contact Person:
Address:	Phone:

Ordering Physician:

Test/Exam Ordered:

Duration:	Do I Need A Driver? YES / NO

Symptoms:

Appt. Date:	Arrival Time ___:___	Exam Time ___:___

Prep For Test:

Results:

Facility:	Contact Person:
Address:	Phone:

Ordering Physician:

Test/Exam Ordered:

Duration:	Do I Need A Driver? YES / NO

Symptoms:

Appt. Date:	Arrival Time ___:___	Exam Time ___:___

Prep For Test:

Results:

MY MEDICAL TESTS/PROCEDURES

Facility: Contact Person:

Address: Phone:

Ordering Physician:

Test/Exam Ordered:

Duration: Do I Need A Driver? YES / NO

Symptoms:

Appt. Date: Arrival Time ___:___   Exam Time ___:___

Prep For Test:

Results:

Facility: Contact Person:

Address: Phone:

Ordering Physician:

Test/Exam Ordered:

Duration: Do I Need A Driver? YES / NO

Symptoms:

Appt. Date: Arrival Time ___:___   Exam Time ___:___

Prep For Test:

Results:

MY MEDICAL TESTS/PROCEDURES

Facility: | Contact Person:

Address: | Phone:

Ordering Physician:

Test/Exam Ordered:

Duration: | Do I Need A Driver? YES / NO

Symptoms:

Appt. Date: | Arrival Time ___:___ | Exam Time ___:___

Prep For Test:

Results:

Facility: | Contact Person:

Address: | Phone:

Ordering Physician:

Test/Exam Ordered:

Duration: | Do I Need A Driver? YES / NO

Symptoms:

Appt. Date: | Arrival Time ___:___ | Exam Time ___:___

Prep For Test:

Results:

MY MEDICAL TESTS/PROCEDURES

Facility: | Contact Person:

Address: | Phone:

Ordering Physician:

Test/Exam Ordered:

Duration: | Do I Need A Driver? YES / NO

Symptoms:

Appt. Date: | Arrival Time ___:___ | Exam Time ___:___

Prep For Test:

Results:

Facility: | Contact Person:

Address: | Phone:

Ordering Physician:

Test/Exam Ordered:

Duration: | Do I Need A Driver? YES / NO

Symptoms:

Appt. Date: | Arrival Time ___:___ | Exam Time ___:___

Prep For Test:

Results:

MY MEDICAL TESTS/PROCEDURES

Facility: | Contact Person:

Address: | Phone:

Ordering Physician:

Test/Exam Ordered:

Duration: | Do I Need A Driver? YES / NO

Symptoms:

Appt. Date: | Arrival Time ___:___ | Exam Time ___:___

Prep For Test:

Results:

Facility: | Contact Person:

Address: | Phone:

Ordering Physician:

Test/Exam Ordered:

Duration: | Do I Need A Driver? YES / NO

Symptoms:

Appt. Date: | Arrival Time ___:___ | Exam Time ___:___

Prep For Test:

Results:

MY MEDICAL TESTS/PROCEDURES

Facility:	Contact Person:
Address:	Phone:
Ordering Physician:	
Test/Exam Ordered:	
Duration:	Do I Need A Driver? YES / NO
Symptoms:	

Appt. Date: _____ Arrival Time ___:___ Exam Time ___:___

Prep For Test:

Results:

Facility:	Contact Person:
Address:	Phone:
Ordering Physician:	
Test/Exam Ordered:	
Duration:	Do I Need A Driver? YES / NO
Symptoms:	

Appt. Date: _____ Arrival Time ___:___ Exam Time ___:___

Prep For Test:

Results:

MY MEDICAL TESTS/PROCEDURES

Facility: Contact Person:

Address: Phone:

Ordering Physician:

Test/Exam Ordered:

Duration: Do I Need A Driver? YES / NO

Symptoms:

Appt. Date: Arrival Time ___:___   Exam Time ___:___

Prep For Test:

Results:

Facility: Contact Person:

Address: Phone:

Ordering Physician:

Test/Exam Ordered:

Duration: Do I Need A Driver? YES / NO

Symptoms:

Appt. Date: Arrival Time ___:___   Exam Time ___:___

Prep For Test:

Results:

MY MEDICAL TESTS/PROCEDURES

Facility: Contact Person:

Address: Phone:

Ordering Physician:

Test/Exam Ordered:

Duration: Do I Need A Driver? YES / NO

Symptoms:

Appt. Date: Arrival Time ___:___   Exam Time ___:___

Prep For Test:

Results:

Facility: Contact Person:

Address: Phone:

Ordering Physician:

Test/Exam Ordered:

Duration: Do I Need A Driver? YES / NO

Symptoms:

Appt. Date: Arrival Time ___:___   Exam Time ___:___

Prep For Test:

Results:

MY MEDICAL TESTS/PROCEDURES

Facility:	Contact Person:
Address:	Phone:
Ordering Physician:	
Test/Exam Ordered:	
Duration:	Do I Need A Driver? YES / NO
Symptoms:	

Appt. Date: | Arrival Time ___:___ | Exam Time ___:___

Prep For Test:

Results:

Facility:	Contact Person:
Address:	Phone:
Ordering Physician:	
Test/Exam Ordered:	
Duration:	Do I Need A Driver? YES / NO
Symptoms:	

Appt. Date: | Arrival Time ___:___ | Exam Time ___:___

Prep For Test:

Results:

MY MEDICAL TESTS/PROCEDURES

Facility: Contact Person:

Address: Phone:

Ordering Physician:

Test/Exam Ordered:

Duration: Do I Need A Driver? YES / NO

Symptoms:

Appt. Date: Arrival Time ___:___   Exam Time ___:___

Prep For Test:

Results:

Facility: Contact Person:

Address: Phone:

Ordering Physician:

Test/Exam Ordered:

Duration: Do I Need A Driver? YES / NO

Symptoms:

Appt. Date: Arrival Time ___:___   Exam Time ___:___

Prep For Test:

Results:

MY MEDICAL TESTS/PROCEDURES

Facility: Contact Person:

Address: Phone:

Ordering Physician:

Test/Exam Ordered:

Duration: Do I Need A Driver? YES / NO

Symptoms:

Appt. Date: Arrival Time ___:___   Exam Time ___:___

Prep For Test:

Results:

Facility: Contact Person:

Address: Phone:

Ordering Physician:

Test/Exam Ordered:

Duration: Do I Need A Driver? YES / NO

Symptoms:

Appt. Date: Arrival Time ___:___   Exam Time ___:___

Prep For Test:

Results:

MY MEDICAL TESTS/PROCEDURES

Facility: Contact Person:

Address: Phone:

Ordering Physician:

Test/Exam Ordered:

Duration: Do I Need A Driver? YES / NO

Symptoms:

Appt. Date: Arrival Time ___:___   Exam Time ___:___

Prep For Test:

Results:

Facility: Contact Person:

Address: Phone:

Ordering Physician:

Test/Exam Ordered:

Duration: Do I Need A Driver? YES / NO

Symptoms:

Appt. Date: Arrival Time ___:___   Exam Time ___:___

Prep For Test:

Results:

MY MEDICAL TESTS/PROCEDURES

Facility:	Contact Person:
Address:	Phone:
Ordering Physician:	
Test/Exam Ordered:	
Duration:	Do I Need A Driver? YES / NO
Symptoms:	

Appt. Date: _____ Arrival Time ___:___ Exam Time ___:___

Prep For Test:

Results:

Facility:	Contact Person:
Address:	Phone:
Ordering Physician:	
Test/Exam Ordered:	
Duration:	Do I Need A Driver? YES / NO
Symptoms:	

Appt. Date: _____ Arrival Time ___:___ Exam Time ___:___

Prep For Test:

Results:

MY MEDICAL TESTS/PROCEDURES

Facility: Contact Person:

Address: Phone:

Ordering Physician:

Test/Exam Ordered:

Duration: Do I Need A Driver? YES / NO

Symptoms:

Appt. Date: Arrival Time ___:___   Exam Time ___:___

Prep For Test:

Results:

Facility: Contact Person:

Address: Phone:

Ordering Physician:

Test/Exam Ordered:

Duration: Do I Need A Driver? YES / NO

Symptoms:

Appt. Date: Arrival Time ___:___   Exam Time ___:___

Prep For Test:

Results:

MY MEDICAL TESTS/PROCEDURES

Facility: | Contact Person:

Address: | Phone:

Ordering Physician:

Test/Exam Ordered:

Duration: | Do I Need A Driver? YES / NO

Symptoms:

Appt. Date: | Arrival Time ___:___ | Exam Time ___:___

Prep For Test:

Results:

Facility: | Contact Person:

Address: | Phone:

Ordering Physician:

Test/Exam Ordered:

Duration: | Do I Need A Driver? YES / NO

Symptoms:

Appt. Date: | Arrival Time ___:___ | Exam Time ___:___

Prep For Test:

Results:

MY MEDICAL TESTS/PROCEDURES

Facility: Contact Person:

Address: Phone:

Ordering Physician:

Test/Exam Ordered:

Duration: Do I Need A Driver? YES / NO

Symptoms:

Appt. Date: Arrival Time ___:___   Exam Time ___:___

Prep For Test:

Results:

Facility: Contact Person:

Address: Phone:

Ordering Physician:

Test/Exam Ordered:

Duration: Do I Need A Driver? YES / NO

Symptoms:

Appt. Date: Arrival Time ___:___   Exam Time ___:___

Prep For Test:

Results:

MY MEDICAL TESTS/PROCEDURES

Facility: | Contact Person:

Address: | Phone:

Ordering Physician:

Test/Exam Ordered:

Duration: | Do I Need A Driver? YES / NO

Symptoms:

Appt. Date: | Arrival Time ___:___ | Exam Time ___:___

Prep For Test:

Results:

Facility: | Contact Person:

Address: | Phone:

Ordering Physician:

Test/Exam Ordered:

Duration: | Do I Need A Driver? YES / NO

Symptoms:

Appt. Date: | Arrival Time ___:___ | Exam Time ___:___

Prep For Test:

Results:

MY MEDICAL TESTS/PROCEDURES

Facility: Contact Person:

Address: Phone:

Ordering Physician:

Test/Exam Ordered:

Duration: Do I Need A Driver? YES / NO

Symptoms:

Appt. Date: Arrival Time ___:___   Exam Time ___:___

Prep For Test:

Results:

Facility: Contact Person:

Address: Phone:

Ordering Physician:

Test/Exam Ordered:

Duration: Do I Need A Driver? YES / NO

Symptoms:

Appt. Date: Arrival Time ___:___   Exam Time ___:___

Prep For Test:

Results:

MY MEDICAL TESTS/PROCEDURES

Facility: | Contact Person:

Address: | Phone:

Ordering Physician:

Test/Exam Ordered:

Duration: | Do I Need A Driver? YES / NO

Symptoms:

Appt. Date: | Arrival Time ___:___ | Exam Time ___:___

Prep For Test:

Results:

Facility: | Contact Person:

Address: | Phone:

Ordering Physician:

Test/Exam Ordered:

Duration: | Do I Need A Driver? YES / NO

Symptoms:

Appt. Date: | Arrival Time ___:___ | Exam Time ___:___

Prep For Test:

Results:

MY MEDICAL TESTS/PROCEDURES

Facility: Contact Person:

Address: Phone:

Ordering Physician:

Test/Exam Ordered:

Duration: Do I Need A Driver? YES / NO

Symptoms:

Appt. Date: Arrival Time ___:___   Exam Time ___:___

Prep For Test:

Results:

Facility: Contact Person:

Address: Phone:

Ordering Physician:

Test/Exam Ordered:

Duration: Do I Need A Driver? YES / NO

Symptoms:

Appt. Date: Arrival Time ___:___   Exam Time ___:___

Prep For Test:

Results:

MY MEDICAL TESTS/PROCEDURES

Facility:	Contact Person:
Address:	Phone:
Ordering Physician:	
Test/Exam Ordered:	
Duration:	Do I Need A Driver? YES / NO
Symptoms:	

Appt. Date:	Arrival Time ___:___	Exam Time ___:___

Prep For Test:

Results:

Facility:	Contact Person:
Address:	Phone:
Ordering Physician:	
Test/Exam Ordered:	
Duration:	Do I Need A Driver? YES / NO
Symptoms:	

Appt. Date:	Arrival Time ___:___	Exam Time ___:___

Prep For Test:

Results:

MY MEDICAL TESTS/PROCEDURES

Facility: Contact Person:

Address: Phone:

Ordering Physician:

Test/Exam Ordered:

Duration: Do I Need A Driver? YES / NO

Symptoms:

Appt. Date: Arrival Time ___:___   Exam Time ___:___

Prep For Test:

Results:

Facility: Contact Person:

Address: Phone:

Ordering Physician:

Test/Exam Ordered:

Duration: Do I Need A Driver? YES / NO

Symptoms:

Appt. Date: Arrival Time ___:___   Exam Time ___:___

Prep For Test:

Results:

MY MEDICAL TESTS/PROCEDURES

Facility:	Contact Person:
Address:	Phone:
Ordering Physician:	
Test/Exam Ordered:	
Duration:	Do I Need A Driver? YES / NO
Symptoms:	

Appt. Date:	Arrival Time ___:___	Exam Time ___:___

Prep For Test:

Results:

Facility:	Contact Person:
Address:	Phone:
Ordering Physician:	
Test/Exam Ordered:	
Duration:	Do I Need A Driver? YES / NO
Symptoms:	

Appt. Date:	Arrival Time ___:___	Exam Time ___:___

Prep For Test:

Results:

MY MEDICAL TESTS/PROCEDURES

Facility:	Contact Person:
Address:	Phone:

Ordering Physician:

Test/Exam Ordered:

Duration:	Do I Need A Driver? YES / NO

Symptoms:

Appt. Date:	Arrival Time ___:___	Exam Time ___:___

Prep For Test:

Results:

Facility:	Contact Person:
Address:	Phone:

Ordering Physician:

Test/Exam Ordered:

Duration:	Do I Need A Driver? YES / NO

Symptoms:

Appt. Date:	Arrival Time ___:___	Exam Time ___:___

Prep For Test:

Results:

MY MEDICAL TESTS/PROCEDURES

Facility: | Contact Person:

Address: | Phone:

Ordering Physician:

Test/Exam Ordered:

Duration: | Do I Need A Driver? YES / NO

Symptoms:

Appt. Date: | Arrival Time ___:___ | Exam Time ___:___

Prep For Test:

Results:

Facility: | Contact Person:

Address: | Phone:

Ordering Physician:

Test/Exam Ordered:

Duration: | Do I Need A Driver? YES / NO

Symptoms:

Appt. Date: | Arrival Time ___:___ | Exam Time ___:___

Prep For Test:

Results:

MY MEDICAL TESTS/PROCEDURES

Facility: Contact Person:

Address: Phone:

Ordering Physician:

Test/Exam Ordered:

Duration: Do I Need A Driver? YES / NO

Symptoms:

Appt. Date: Arrival Time ___:___   Exam Time ___:___

Prep For Test:

Results:

Facility: Contact Person:

Address: Phone:

Ordering Physician:

Test/Exam Ordered:

Duration: Do I Need A Driver? YES / NO

Symptoms:

Appt. Date: Arrival Time ___:___   Exam Time ___:___

Prep For Test:

Results:

MY MEDICAL TESTS/PROCEDURES

Facility: Contact Person:

Address: Phone:

Ordering Physician:

Test/Exam Ordered:

Duration: Do I Need A Driver? YES / NO

Symptoms:

Appt. Date: Arrival Time ___:___   Exam Time ___:___

Prep For Test:

Results:

Facility: Contact Person:

Address: Phone:

Ordering Physician:

Test/Exam Ordered:

Duration: Do I Need A Driver? YES / NO

Symptoms:

Appt. Date: Arrival Time ___:___   Exam Time ___:___

Prep For Test:

Results:

MY MEDICAL TESTS/PROCEDURES

Facility: Contact Person:

Address: Phone:

Ordering Physician:

Test/Exam Ordered:

Duration: Do I Need A Driver? YES / NO

Symptoms:

Appt. Date: Arrival Time ___:___   Exam Time ___:___

Prep For Test:

Results:

Facility: Contact Person:

Address: Phone:

Ordering Physician:

Test/Exam Ordered:

Duration: Do I Need A Driver? YES / NO

Symptoms:

Appt. Date: Arrival Time ___:___   Exam Time ___:___

Prep For Test:

Results:

MY MEDICAL TESTS/PROCEDURES

Facility: Contact Person:

Address: Phone:

Ordering Physician:

Test/Exam Ordered:

Duration: Do I Need A Driver? YES / NO

Symptoms:

Appt. Date: Arrival Time ___:___   Exam Time ___:___

Prep For Test:

Results:

Facility: Contact Person:

Address: Phone:

Ordering Physician:

Test/Exam Ordered:

Duration: Do I Need A Driver? YES / NO

Symptoms:

Appt. Date: Arrival Time ___:___   Exam Time ___:___

Prep For Test:

Results:

MY MEDICAL TESTS/PROCEDURES

Facility:	Contact Person:
Address:	Phone:

Ordering Physician:

Test/Exam Ordered:

Duration:	Do I Need A Driver? YES / NO

Symptoms:

Appt. Date:	Arrival Time ___:___	Exam Time ___:___

Prep For Test:

Results:

Facility:	Contact Person:
Address:	Phone:

Ordering Physician:

Test/Exam Ordered:

Duration:	Do I Need A Driver? YES / NO

Symptoms:

Appt. Date:	Arrival Time ___:___	Exam Time ___:___

Prep For Test:

Results:

MY MEDICAL TESTS/PROCEDURES

Facility:	Contact Person:
Address:	Phone:
Ordering Physician:	
Test/Exam Ordered:	
Duration:	Do I Need A Driver? YES / NO
Symptoms:	

Appt. Date:	Arrival Time ___:___	Exam Time ___:___

Prep For Test:

Results:

Facility:	Contact Person:
Address:	Phone:
Ordering Physician:	
Test/Exam Ordered:	
Duration:	Do I Need A Driver? YES / NO
Symptoms:	

Appt. Date:	Arrival Time ___:___	Exam Time ___:___

Prep For Test:

Results:

MY MEDICAL TESTS/PROCEDURES

Facility: | Contact Person:

Address: | Phone:

Ordering Physician:

Test/Exam Ordered:

Duration: | Do I Need A Driver? YES / NO

Symptoms:

Appt. Date: | Arrival Time ___:___ | Exam Time ___:___

Prep For Test:

Results:

Facility: | Contact Person:

Address: | Phone:

Ordering Physician:

Test/Exam Ordered:

Duration: | Do I Need A Driver? YES / NO

Symptoms:

Appt. Date: | Arrival Time ___:___ | Exam Time ___:___

Prep For Test:

Results:

MY MEDICAL TESTS/PROCEDURES

Facility:	Contact Person:
Address:	Phone:
Ordering Physician:	
Test/Exam Ordered:	
Duration:	Do I Need A Driver? YES / NO
Symptoms:	

Appt. Date: _____ Arrival Time ___:___ Exam Time ___:___

Prep For Test:

Results:

Facility:	Contact Person:
Address:	Phone:
Ordering Physician:	
Test/Exam Ordered:	
Duration:	Do I Need A Driver? YES / NO
Symptoms:	

Appt. Date: _____ Arrival Time ___:___ Exam Time ___:___

Prep For Test:

Results:

MY MEDICAL TESTS/PROCEDURES

Facility:	Contact Person:
Address:	Phone:
Ordering Physician:	
Test/Exam Ordered:	
Duration:	Do I Need A Driver? YES / NO
Symptoms:	

Appt. Date: Arrival Time ___:___   Exam Time ___:___

Prep For Test:

Results:

Facility:	Contact Person:
Address:	Phone:
Ordering Physician:	
Test/Exam Ordered:	
Duration:	Do I Need A Driver? YES / NO
Symptoms:	

Appt. Date: Arrival Time ___:___   Exam Time ___:___

Prep For Test:

Results:

MY MEDICAL TESTS/PROCEDURES

Facility: Contact Person:

Address: Phone:

Ordering Physician:

Test/Exam Ordered:

Duration: Do I Need A Driver? YES / NO

Symptoms:

Appt. Date: Arrival Time ___:___   Exam Time ___:___

Prep For Test:

Results:

Facility: Contact Person:

Address: Phone:

Ordering Physician:

Test/Exam Ordered:

Duration: Do I Need A Driver? YES / NO

Symptoms:

Appt. Date: Arrival Time ___:___   Exam Time ___:___

Prep For Test:

Results:

MY MEDICAL TESTS/PROCEDURES

Facility:	Contact Person:
Address:	Phone:

Ordering Physician:

Test/Exam Ordered:

Duration:	Do I Need A Driver? YES / NO

Symptoms:

Appt. Date:	Arrival Time ___:___	Exam Time ___:___

Prep For Test:

Results:

Facility:	Contact Person:
Address:	Phone:

Ordering Physician:

Test/Exam Ordered:

Duration:	Do I Need A Driver? YES / NO

Symptoms:

Appt. Date:	Arrival Time ___:___	Exam Time ___:___

Prep For Test:

Results:

MY MEDICAL TESTS/PROCEDURES

Facility: Contact Person:

Address: Phone:

Ordering Physician:

Test/Exam Ordered:

Duration: Do I Need A Driver? YES / NO

Symptoms:

Appt. Date: Arrival Time ___:___   Exam Time ___:___

Prep For Test:

Results:

Facility: Contact Person:

Address: Phone:

Ordering Physician:

Test/Exam Ordered:

Duration: Do I Need A Driver? YES / NO

Symptoms:

Appt. Date: Arrival Time ___:___   Exam Time ___:___

Prep For Test:

Results:

MY MEDICAL TESTS/PROCEDURES

Facility:	Contact Person:
Address:	Phone:

Ordering Physician:

Test/Exam Ordered:

Duration:	Do I Need A Driver? YES / NO

Symptoms:

Appt. Date:	Arrival Time ___:___	Exam Time ___:___

Prep For Test:

Results:

Facility:	Contact Person:
Address:	Phone:

Ordering Physician:

Test/Exam Ordered:

Duration:	Do I Need A Driver? YES / NO

Symptoms:

Appt. Date:	Arrival Time ___:___	Exam Time ___:___

Prep For Test:

Results:

MY MEDICAL TESTS/PROCEDURES

Facility:	Contact Person:
Address:	Phone:
Ordering Physician:	
Test/Exam Ordered:	
Duration:	Do I Need A Driver? YES / NO
Symptoms:	

Appt. Date: _____ Arrival Time ___:___ Exam Time ___:___

Prep For Test:

Results:

Facility:	Contact Person:
Address:	Phone:
Ordering Physician:	
Test/Exam Ordered:	
Duration:	Do I Need A Driver? YES / NO
Symptoms:	

Appt. Date: _____ Arrival Time ___:___ Exam Time ___:___

Prep For Test:

Results:

MY MEDICAL TESTS/PROCEDURES

Facility: Contact Person:

Address: Phone:

Ordering Physician:

Test/Exam Ordered:

Duration: Do I Need A Driver? YES / NO

Symptoms:

Appt. Date: Arrival Time ___:___   Exam Time ___:___

Prep For Test:

Results:

Facility: Contact Person:

Address: Phone:

Ordering Physician:

Test/Exam Ordered:

Duration: Do I Need A Driver? YES / NO

Symptoms:

Appt. Date: Arrival Time ___:___   Exam Time ___:___

Prep For Test:

Results:

MY MEDICAL TESTS/PROCEDURES

Facility:	Contact Person:
Address:	Phone:
Ordering Physician:	
Test/Exam Ordered:	
Duration:	Do I Need A Driver? YES / NO
Symptoms:	

Appt. Date: Arrival Time ___:___   Exam Time ___:___

Prep For Test:

Results:

Facility:	Contact Person:
Address:	Phone:
Ordering Physician:	
Test/Exam Ordered:	
Duration:	Do I Need A Driver? YES / NO
Symptoms:	

Appt. Date: Arrival Time ___:___   Exam Time ___:___

Prep For Test:

Results:

MY MEDICAL TESTS/PROCEDURES

Facility: Contact Person:

Address: Phone:

Ordering Physician:

Test/Exam Ordered:

Duration: Do I Need A Driver? YES / NO

Symptoms:

Appt. Date: Arrival Time ___:___   Exam Time ___:___

Prep For Test:

Results:

Facility: Contact Person:

Address: Phone:

Ordering Physician:

Test/Exam Ordered:

Duration: Do I Need A Driver? YES / NO

Symptoms:

Appt. Date: Arrival Time ___:___   Exam Time ___:___

Prep For Test:

Results:

MY MEDICAL TESTS/PROCEDURES

Facility: Contact Person:

Address: Phone:

Ordering Physician:

Test/Exam Ordered:

Duration: Do I Need A Driver? YES / NO

Symptoms:

Appt. Date: Arrival Time ___:___   Exam Time ___:___

Prep For Test:

Results:

Facility: Contact Person:

Address: Phone:

Ordering Physician:

Test/Exam Ordered:

Duration: Do I Need A Driver? YES / NO

Symptoms:

Appt. Date: Arrival Time ___:___   Exam Time ___:___

Prep For Test:

Results: